"Sugar-Free Success: A Flavorful Guide to Diabetic Cooking and Meal Planning"

Allison W. Archer

"Sugar-Free Success: A Flavorful Guide to Diabetic Cooking and Meal Planning"

Table of Content

Introduction

"Sugar-Free Success" is pleased to welcome you. I hope that while you navigate the world of diabetes care and adopt a healthy lifestyle through scrumptious, balanced meals, this book will serve as your dependable guide.

Finding out you have diabetes can be stressful and raise a lot of questions and worries. I know starting a new diet can be intimidating, but don't worry—you're not the only one. This book is here to help you every step of the way, offering insightful advice, useful tips, and delectable recipes adapted to your dietary requirements.

I'll go through the basics of diabetes in this introduction, such as its types, causes, and symptoms. Making educated choices regarding your nutrition and general well being requires having a thorough understanding of your situation. I'll explain how a diabetic-friendly diet

4

can improve your health and give you the power to decide how you want to live your life.

The chapters in this book discuss many facets of diabetic meal preparation and cooking. I'll start by providing you with the basic essentials you'll need to prepare wholesome, nourishing meals. We'll work together to fill your pantry with diabetic-friendly essentials so you have everything you need close at hand.

Diabetes management requires careful meal planning, which I will walk you through. The essentials of diabetic meal preparation, such as portion control and carbohydrate tracking, will be revealed. I'll offer helpful advice on putting together balanced plates that help control blood sugar levels and advance general wellness.

As the most crucial meal of the day, breakfast, I've gathered a collection of stimulating and simple breakfast recipes. You can choose from a variety of delectable breakfast selections to get your day started, ranging from quick and filling options to grab-and-go breakfasts for those hectic mornings.

It is possible to have a variety of filling and nutritious meals during lunch. We will look at a range of recipes together to find something that you would enjoy. My lunch recipes range from colorful salads to filling soups and stews, all of which are meant to keep you full and energized all day.

I realize how important it is to have supper options that are tasty, healthy, and simple to make. My supper recipes cover a wide range of cuisines, from one-pot dinners ideal for hectic weeknights to vegetarian and vegan options that satisfy various dietary needs.

For people with diabetes, snacks and appetizers might occasionally be difficult, but I think that snacking can still be pleasurable and nutritious. You may find my clever snacking suggestions and delectable appetizer dishes in this book, which will satisfy you in between meals and wow your guests at parties.

Desserts haven't been forgotten, of course! You may enjoy sweets guilt-free thanks to a selection of diabetic-friendly delicacies I've put up. You'll learn that having diabetes doesn't mean you have to give up enjoying a sweet pleasure, from light and refreshing options to delicious desserts with healthy twists.

You can use the meal plans and sample meals offered to help you on your quest for better diabetes management. These menus give options for various seasons and holidays and cater to diverse calorie needs. I'll also offer advice on how to eat out while still sticking to a diabetic-friendly diet.

Making lifestyle decisions that support your general wellbeing is an important part of managing diabetes. We will discuss how physical activity, stress reduction, and exercise can all help with diabetes management.

Additionally, I'll give you access to tools for additional learning and support so you may succeed on your diabetic journey.

This book is filled with useful advice, professional suggestions, and more than a hundred mouthwatering diabetic-friendly recipes. My intention is to motivate you to adopt a balanced, healthy lifestyle while still appreciating the delights of food.

Keep in mind that we are on a journey of empowerment and self-discovery. You have the ability to take charge of your health and wellbeing by practicing thoughtful decision-making and adopting a diabetic-friendly diet. This book isn't just about limitations; it's also about discovering new flavors, learning inventive cooking methods, and taking pleasure in feeding your body.

I am familiar with the feelings and doubts that might accompany this path because I have first-hand experience with the difficulties that come with being diagnosed with diabetes. However, I want to reassure you that managing diabetes may become second nature if you have the correct information and assistance.

I'll offer my own experiences, useful advice, and lessons learnt throughout this book to help you get over any obstacles you may run into. I advise you to enter this new phase of your life with an open mind and the readiness to try new things in the kitchen. Accept the chance to learn about new flavors, ingredients, and culinary customs that will not only improve your health but also broaden your culinary horizons.

Keep in mind that this book is intended exclusively for people who have just received a diabetes diagnosis. I'll provide you the fundamental information you need to choose your diet and way of life wisely. I'm here to help you every step of the way, from comprehending how carbohydrates affect blood sugar levels to deciphering food labels and portion sizes.

Although this book is a comprehensive reference, it is still important to seek the advice and suggestions of a certified dietician or your healthcare professional. They will be able to offer insightful advice suited to your particular requirements and situation.

I want to remind you to be patient and nice to yourself as we travel this path together. It takes time and effort to become accustomed to a new dietary routine and manage diabetes. Keep in mind that making little, regular changes can have a big impact on your health over the long term.

I'm thrilled to be a part of your diabetic journey, and I really think that you can have a happy, active life despite having diabetes if you have access to the correct information, encouragement, and delectable recipes. So let's explore the world of diabetic meal planning and cooking and seize this chance to feed our bodies and care for our wellbeing.

The "Sugar-Free Success" is your guide to a delicious, healthy, and empowering journey.

Chapter 1

Understanding Diabetes: Types, Causes, and Symptoms

Diabetes is a chronic illness that affects millions of people throughout the world. It is defined by the body's inability to control blood sugar levels effectively, which results in increased blood glucose levels. Understanding the different forms, causes, and symptoms of diabetes is crucial for managing disease well and for making educated decisions about nutrition and lifestyle.

Diabetes Types

Diabetes comes in a variety of forms, each with its own characteristics and causes. The most typical varieties include:

1. Type 1 Diabetes: In this kind of diabetes, the pancreatic insulin-producing cells are wrongly

12

attacked and destroyed by the immune system. A lifelong reliance on insulin shots results from the body's inability to create enough insulin.

2. Type 2 Diabetes: Type 2 diabetes is the most common type and is frequently linked to sedentary lifestyles, obesity, and poor eating habits. In this case, the body either stops producing enough insulin or develops an insulin resistance that makes it difficult to keep blood sugar levels normal.

3. Gestational Diabetes: Approximately 2-10% of pregnant women develop gestational diabetes during their pregnancy. High blood sugar levels that start during pregnancy and usually go away after giving delivery are its defining features. Women who experienced gestational diabetes, on the other hand, are more likely to develop type 2 diabetes later in life.

Diabetes Causes

Although the precise origins of diabetes are not entirely understood, a number of things can lead to its occurrence:

1. Genetic Propensity: Having a family history of diabetes can make you more likely to have the disease. Although other factors, including as lifestyle decisions, also play an important influence, some genes can increase a person's susceptibility to diabetes.

2. Obesity and Lifestyle Factors: Type 2 diabetes is significantly increased by excess body weight, especially in the abdomen. Diabetes can develop as a result of unhealthy eating patterns, inactivity, and sedentary lifestyles.

3. Autoimmune Response: In type 1 diabetes, the immune system unintentionally targets and kills the pancreatic cells that make insulin. Although the precise causes of this autoimmune reaction are still under investigation, it is thought to be a result of a combination of hereditary and environmental factors.

Diabetes Symptoms

For early detection and intervention, it is essential to be able to recognize the signs of diabetes. Diabetic symptoms frequently manifest as:

1. Increased urination: One of the first apparent signs of diabetes is frequently increased urine. The frequency of urination rises as a result of the kidneys having to work harder to filter and absorb more blood sugar.

2. Excessive thirst: Dehydration brought on by increased urine can result in excessive thirst.

3. Unexplained weight loss: People with untreated diabetes who cannot adequately use glucose as an energy source may experience unexplained weight loss.

4. Weakness and exhaustion: Low insulin levels or insulin resistance can prevent glucose from entering cells, resulting in a sensation of weakness and fatigue.

5. Slow wound healing: High blood sugar levels might hinder the body's capacity to adequately repair wounds, resulting in a delayed healing.

6. Blurred vision: High blood sugar levels can harm the eye's lens, impairing eyesight.

7. Numbness or tingling in the extremities: High blood sugar levels over time can harm nerves, causing tingling or numbness, especially in the hands and feet.

Having a Diabetic-Friendly Diet is Important

Effective diabetes management depends on eating a well-balanced, diabetic-friendly diet. It boosts general health, lowers the risk of problems, and aids in blood sugar regulation.

Here are some main arguments in favor of diabetic-friendly eating:

1. Blood sugar control is the main goal of a diabetic-friendly diet, which also balances carbohydrates with proteins and healthy fats. As a result, blood sugar levels are better controlled and spikes and crashes that could be harmful to general health are avoided. People with diabetes can better manage their health and reduce the need for insulin or medication by making informed decisions about the types and amounts of carbs they consume.

2. **Control of weight:** To effectively manage diabetes, a healthy weight must be maintained. A diet that is suitable for people with diabetes stresses portion management, promotes the consumption of nutrient-dense meals, and restricts the consumption of foods that are high in sugar, bad fats, and empty calories. A diabetic-friendly diet can boost metabolic health and insulin sensitivity by encouraging weight loss or weight maintenance.

3. Cardiovascular Health: Diabetes and an increased risk of cardiovascular diseases are closely related. By enhancing blood pressure, cholesterol levels, and cardiovascular health, a diabetic-friendly diet high in whole grains, lean proteins, fruits, vegetables, and healthy fats can help lower the risk of heart disease.

4. Nutritional Adequacy: Diabetes need not prevent you from consuming a wide range of delectable and healthy foods. A carefully thought-out diabetic-friendly diet can include all the vital vitamins, minerals, and nutrients required for optimum health. People with diabetes can ensure they achieve their nutritional needs while controlling their blood sugar levels by ingesting a variety of foods.

5. Prevention of Long-Term issues: Adhering to a diabetic-friendly diet regularly will assist to stop or delay the emergence of long-term issues related to diabetes. These side effects include circulation problems, kidney disorders, vision issues, and nerve damage. A balanced diet can help people lower the risk of these issues and enhance their overall quality of life by helping them maintain stable blood sugar levels.

How to Benefit from This Book

The comprehensive resource "Sugar-Free Success" was created especially for people who have just received a diabetes diagnosis. My goal is to arm you with the information, resources, and delectable recipes required to successfully navigate your new nutritional adventure.

This book provides a wealth of knowledge about diabetic meal planning and cooking, giving you the practical advice you need to make educated decisions about your diet. It addresses important subjects such pantry essentials, menu planning techniques, portion control, and carbohydrate tracking. With this information, you will be able to prepare meals that are nutritious and well-balanced and that will promote your overall health.

Breakfast, lunch, dinner, snacks, and desserts are just a few of the mealtimes covered in the book's several chapters. A selection of delectable recipes that are adapted to the needs of people with diabetes are provided in each chapter. These recipes have undergone rigorous development to make sure they are tasty, filling, and simple to make.

This book includes recipes as well as meal plans and example menus to assist you in beginning your diabetic-friendly journey. These menus give options for various seasons and holidays and cater to diverse calorie needs. You can make meal planning easier and enjoy a wide variety of foods while successfully controlling your diabetes by using these meal plans.

In addition, this book contains more than just menu ideas and recipes. It explores the significance of physical activity, stress reduction, and lifestyle decisions in the management of diabetes. It gives advice on how to incorporate exercise into your daily routine as well as suggestions for handling social situations and eating out while following a diabetic-friendly diet.

You will develop the self-assurance and abilities necessary to take charge of your diabetes and adopt a healthier, more meaningful lifestyle by adopting the information and useful practices discussed in this book into your daily life.

Chapter 2

Essential Tools and Ingredients

Having the correct tools and supplies in your kitchen can make all the difference when going on a diabetic-friendly culinary journey. This section will walk you through the necessary kitchen equipment for diabetes cooking as well as the ingredients you must have in your diabetic pantry. Having these ingredients on hand will allow you to cook delicious, nutritious meals while successfully managing your diabetes.

Cooking Equipment for Diabetics

1. Measuring Cups and Spoons: In diabetic cooking, precise portion management is essential. Purchase a set of measuring cups and spoons to verify that you are using the exact proportions of components, especially carbs.

2. Food Scale: A food scale is a crucial tool for exact measurement, especially for portioning protein sources and measuring products with different carbohydrate levels.

3. Nonstick Cookware: Because nonstick pans and pots require little oil or fat to cook with, they are great for producing healthy, low-fat meals. They also make cleanup easier because they require less scrubbing.

4. Steamer Basket: Steaming vegetables helps them retain nutrients while adding no extra fat or calories. A steamer basket is a simple and practical instrument for perfectly preparing vegetables.

5. Slow Cooker or Crockpot: A slow cooker is a useful gadget for busy people. It enables you to make delectable dishes with little effort. It's especially great for cooking lean meats, beans, and stews, which are good for diabetics.

6. Blender or Food Processor: These multipurpose equipment are great for producing healthy smoothies, soups, sauces, and dips. They enable you to make healthful, home-cooked substitutes for store-bought products that may have additional sweets or unhealthy additives.

7. Grater and Zester: A grater and zester can be used to add flavor bursts to foods without adding too much salt or sugar. They can be used to grate fresh garlic, ginger, or citrus zest to add flavor to your dishes.

8. Oven Thermometer: An oven thermometer guarantees that your oven is properly calibrated, allowing you to cook at precise temperatures. When baking diabetic-friendly foods and roasting proteins, this is very important.

Essential Diabetic Pantry Ingredients

1. Whole Grains: Choose whole grains like quinoa, brown rice, whole wheat pasta, and

rolled oats. These contain more fiber, vitamins, and minerals than refined foods and have a lower influence on blood sugar levels.

2. Legumes: Beans, lentils, and chickpeas are high in plant protein and fiber. They can be used in soups, stews, salads, and as a meat substitute in some dishes.

3. Lean Proteins: Stock your cupboard with lean protein sources such as skinless poultry, fish, tofu, and lentils. These protein-rich options are lower in saturated fat, making them healthier options for diabetics.

4. Fresh Fruits and veggies: Keep a variety of fresh fruits and veggies in your cupboard and refrigerator. These nutrient-dense meals are abundant in fiber, vitamins, and minerals while being low in calories. They enhance the flavor, texture, and color of your food.

5. Healthy Fats: Choose healthy fat sources such as olive oil, avocado oil, nuts, and seeds. These

fats aid in the absorption of fat-soluble vitamins, increase satiety, and improve heart health.

6. Herbs and spices: Keep a variety of herbs and spices on hand to add flavor to your foods without relying on too much salt or sugar. To improve the flavor of your dishes, experiment with seasonings such as cinnamon, turmeric, cumin, and oregano.

7. Low Sodium Condiments: Choose low-sodium condiments such as reduced-sodium soy sauce, vinegar, mustard, and herb and spice blends that do not contain added salt. These can give your dishes more depth and taste without drastically raising your sodium intake.

8. Sugar replacements: To satisfy your sweet tooth without affecting your blood sugar levels, keep sugar replacements on hand, such as stevia, erythritol, or monk fruit sweetener. They can be used in baking, beverages, and other sweetening dishes.

9. Canned products: Select canned products with reduced sodium or no salt added, such as diced tomatoes, tomato sauce, beans, and broth. These are pantry basics that may be used as soup, stew, and sauce bases, adding fiber and flavor to your dishes.

10. Nutritional Labels: When purchasing packaged foods, pay attention to nutritional labels. Look for items with reduced levels of sugar, sodium, and saturated fat. Reading labels can assist you in making informed decisions and selecting goods that are compatible with your diabetes diet plan.

11. Sugar-free or unsweetened beverages, such as herbal teas, infused water, and sugar-free drink mixes, should be kept on hand. Staying hydrated is important for overall health and can aid in the regulation of cravings and blood sugar levels.

12. Emergency Snacks: Having emergency snacks on hand is a good idea for those times

when you need a quick bite. Choose low-sugar options such as nuts, seeds, nut butter, whole grain crackers, or protein bars for diabetics.

By stocking up on diabetic-friendly foods and equipping your kitchen with these important equipment, you'll be well-prepared to cook delicious and balanced meals that support your diabetes control. To have a well-rounded assortment of nutritional options, check expiration dates on a regular basis and replace your pantry as needed. You'll have the foundation for effective diabetic cooking and a healthy lifestyle if you have these things on hand.

Chapter 3

Meal Planning Fundamentals

Meal planning is an important part of effectively managing diabetes. It entails careful consideration of the items you eat, portion sizes, and meal balancing in order to maintain stable blood sugar levels. This part will go through the essentials of diabetic meal planning, such as portion control, carbohydrate counting, and building a balanced plate to help you achieve your overall health and diabetes management goals.

1. Recognizing Portion Control:

Portion control is critical for diabetics to manage blood sugar levels and maintain a healthy weight. It entails being attentive of the amount of food you consume. Here are some ways to practice portion control:

- Use measuring cups and spoons to measure out foods, especially carbs, which can have a substantial impact on blood sugar levels.

- Learn how to estimate appropriate portion proportions using visual cues. A meal of protein, for example, should be about the size of your palm, a serving of grains or starchy vegetables should be about the size of your cupped hand, and a serving of fats should be about the size of your thumb.

- When dining out or eating pre-packaged meals, keep portion proportions in mind. Because restaurants frequently provide larger servings, consider splitting a meal or ordering a takeout box to divide out half of your meal before you begin eating.

- Slow down and engage in mindful eating. To avoid overeating and promote a better understanding of portion sizes that fulfill your desire without excess, pay attention to hunger and fullness cues.

2. Counting Carbohydrates:

Carbohydrate counting is an important method for regulating blood sugar levels since carbs have the greatest impact on blood glucose levels. It entails keeping track of the amount of carbs you ingest at each meal and, if necessary, balancing it with appropriate insulin or medicine doses. Here are some carbohydrate counting tips:

- Recognize carbohydrate sources in your meals, such as grains, fruits, starchy vegetables, legumes, and dairy products. These food groups are the subject of carbohydrate counting.
- In order to discover the total carbs per serving in packaged foods, read the nutrition labels. To precisely count your carbohydrate intake, pay attention to portion sizes.
- Track your carbohydrate intake with a meal diary or a mobile app. This can assist you in identifying patterns, making changes, and maintaining consistency in your food planning.
- Consult a registered dietitian or a certified diabetes educator to determine an optimal carbohydrate intake range based on your specific

needs, activity levels, and diabetes management goals.

3. Putting Together a Balanced Plate:

Creating a balanced plate is critical for achieving appropriate nutrition and keeping blood sugar levels consistent. It entails incorporating a range of food groups and being mindful of portion sizes. Here's how a balanced dish looks:

- Make half of your plate non-starchy veggies, such as leafy greens, broccoli, peppers, or cucumbers. These are high in vitamins, minerals, and fiber while being low in carbs.
- Reserve a quarter of your plate for lean proteins like skinless chicken, fish, tofu, or lentils. These supply vital amino acids for muscle repair and aid in blood sugar regulation.
- The remaining quarter of your plate should be filled with whole grains or starchy vegetables such as quinoa, brown rice, sweet potatoes, or whole wheat bread. These are carbohydrate sources that provide long-lasting energy.

- Include a little amount of healthy fats such as olive oil, avocados, almonds, or seeds. These help with satiety, heart health, and the absorption of fat-soluble vitamins.
- To enhance general health and digestion, pair your balanced plate with a source of hydration such as water, unsweetened tea, or infused water.

When constructing your balanced meal, keep in mind individual nutritional demands, medication requirements, and personal preferences. Review and change your meal plan on a regular basis based on your blood sugar levels, weight loss objectives, and any advice from your healthcare team. Here are some other meal planning suggestions:

- Strive for diversity: Include a variety of colorful fruits and vegetables, lean meats, whole grains, and healthy fats in your meals. This guarantees a varied range of nutrients while also keeping your meals interesting and pleasurable.
- Be cautious of portion sizes: Portion management should be practiced not only for

carbohydrates but also for proteins and lipids. Use smaller plates or bowls to give the appearance of a fuller plate while eating proper servings.

- Plan for snacks: Include healthy snack options in your meal plan to maintain stable blood sugar levels throughout the day. Choose snacks that contain protein, fiber, and healthy fats to deliver long-lasting energy and satiety.

- Meal prep and batch cooking: Make time for meal preparation and batch cooking to make your week easier. Preparing meals and snacks ahead of time allows you to have nutritious options easily available, saving time and minimizing your reliance on less healthy options.

- Pay attention to your body: Notice how certain foods affect your blood sugar levels, energy levels, and overall well-being. Everyone's reaction to food is different, so pay attention to how specific foods or combinations make you feel.

- Seek help: Consider joining a diabetes support group or interacting with other diabetics. Sharing experiences, exchanging ideas, and receiving encouragement can be extremely beneficial on your path to better health.

You may take charge of your nutrition, effectively manage your blood sugar levels, and promote overall well-being by knowing the foundations of diabetic meal planning, practicing portion control and carbohydrate counting, and making balanced plates. Remember that consistency and individualization are essential in determining the ideal food plan for you. You may build a sustainable and enjoyable approach to diabetes meal planning that supports your long-term health objectives with time, patience, and the advice of healthcare specialists.

Chapter 4

Breakfast Recipes

Breakfast is widely regarded as the most essential meal of the day since it gives you with the energy and nutrition you need to start your day off well. Breakfast options that help diabetics maintain stable blood sugar levels and support overall health are crucial. In this section, we'll look at a variety of breakfast recipes, including energizing options to start your day, quick and easy diabetic-friendly breakfasts, and convenient grab-and-go options.

1. Energizing Breakfasts to Start Your Day:

a) Vegetable Omelet: 2 large eggs
- 1/4 cup chopped bell peppers
1/4 cup chopped onions
- 1 tablespoon fresh herbs, chopped (parsley, chives, etc.)

- Season to suit with salt and pepper - Cooking spray

Instructions:
1. Whisk together the eggs in a mixing dish and season with salt and pepper.
2. Spray a nonstick skillet lightly with cooking spray and heat over medium heat.
3. Cook the diced bell peppers, onions, and mushrooms in the skillet until tender.
4. Pour the beaten eggs over the vegetables and cook until the eggs are set.
5. Before folding the omelet in half, garnish with fresh herbs.
6. Arrange on a plate and serve.

c) Greek Yogurt Parfait:
Ingredients:
- 1/2 cup plain Greek yogurt
1/4 cup fresh berries (strawberries, blueberries, raspberries, and so on)
- 2 tablespoons chopped nuts or seeds (almonds, walnuts, chia seeds)

- 1 tbsp honey or sugar streusel-a sugar-free sweetener is optional.

Instructions:
1. In a glass or bowl, layer the Greek yogurt, fresh berries, and chopped nuts or seeds.
2. Drizzle with honey or a sugar-free sweetener if desired.
3. Serve right away or chill overnight for a great grab-and-go option.

2. Quick and Easy Diabetic Breakfasts:

Overnight Chia Pudding: - 2 tablespoons chia seeds
- 1/2 cup unsweetened almond milk (or other preferred milk)
- 1 teaspoon vanilla extract
- Optional garnishes include fresh fruit or almonds.

Instructions:

1. In a jar or container, combine the chia seeds, almond milk, and vanilla essence. Stir everything together completely.
2. Cover and refrigerate overnight.
3. In the morning, give it a good stir and top with fresh fruit or nuts if desired for more flavor and texture.
4. Enjoy the creamy, healthy chia pudding.

b) Avocado Toast: 1 piece whole grain bread - half an avocado, mashed
- Squeeze lemon juice
- A teaspoon of salt and pepper to taste - Optional garnishes include sliced tomato, feta cheese, and a poached egg.

1. Toast the whole wheat bread till crisp.
2. In a small bowl, mash the avocado with the lemon juice, salt, and pepper.
3. Arrange the toasted bread on top of the avocado.
4. Top with your chosen garnishes.
5. Serve immediately for a quick and satisfying breakfast.

3. On-the-Go Breakfast Options:

a) Breakfast Muffins: - 1 cup almond flour - 1/2 cup rolled oats - 1/4 cup unsweetened applesauce - 2 tablespoons honey or sugar substitute-no sweetness
- 2 eggs
1 tbsp. baking powder
- 1/2 teaspoon cinnamon powder
- 1/4 teaspoon salt - 1/2 cup chopped fresh fruit (apples or berries)
- 1/4 cup chopped nuts (preferably walnuts or almonds)

1. Preheat the oven to 350 degrees Fahrenheit/175 degrees Celsius and line a muffin tray with paper liners.
2. In a large mixing bowl, combine almond flour, rolled oats, baking powder, cinnamon, and salt.
3. In a separate bowl, whisk together applesauce, honey, and eggs until completely combined.
4. Combine the wet and dry ingredients in a mixing bowl until just combined.

5. Fold in the fresh fruit and almonds.
6. Divide the batter evenly between the muffin cups, filling them about three-quarters full.
7. Bake the cake for 18-20 minutes, or until a toothpick inserted into the center comes out clean.
8. Before transferring the muffins to a wire rack to finish cooling, give them a few minutes to cool in the pan.
9. Store the muffins in an airtight container in the refrigerator for easy breakfasts throughout the week.

b) Protein Smoothie
1 cup unsweetened almond milk (or other milk of choice)
- 1/2 cup plain Greek yogurt
- 1 scoop protein powder (preferably low-sugar)
- 1 tablespoon nut butter (recommended almond or peanut butter)
- 1 frozen banana or 1 cup frozen berries
- Add a handful of spinach or kale for extra nourishment.

Instructions:

1. In a blender, combine almond milk, Greek yogurt, protein powder, nut butter, and frozen berries or banana.

2. Add a handful of spinach or kale for extra greens.

3. Continue blending the mixture until it is creamy and smooth.

4. Transfer to a portable cup or bottle and enjoy.

5. Refrigerate it and give it a quick shake before serving if you made it ahead of time.

These breakfast recipes offer a variety of options to fit your tastes and hectic mornings. There's a breakfast meal for everyone, whether you have time to make a robust omelet, prefer quick and easy options like overnight chia pudding or avocado toast, or require a practical grab-and-go option like breakfast muffins or a protein smoothie. Begin your day with a substantial and diabetic-friendly breakfast that will set the tone for the rest of your day.

Here are a few additional breakfast options to spice up your diabetic-friendly eating plan:

1. Breakfast Burrito with Eggs and Vegetables:

Ingredients:
- 1 whole grain tortilla
- 2 big scrambled eggs
- 1/4 cup bell peppers, diced
- 1/4 cup chopped onions
- 1/4 cup thinly sliced mushrooms
- 1/4 cup low-fat shredded cheese
- Season with salt and pepper to taste - Serve with salsa or hot sauce (optional).

Instructions:
1. Sauté the bell peppers, onions, and mushrooms in a nonstick skillet until soft.
2. Cook the scrambled eggs in the skillet until done.
3. Top with the shredded cheese and heat until melted.

4. Microwave or warm the tortilla in a separate skillet.

5. Spread the egg and veggie mixture onto a tortilla, roll it up, and serve with salsa or hot sauce, if preferred.

2. Quinoa Breakfast Bowl:

Combine the following ingredients:
- 1/4 cup plain Greek yogurt - 1/2 cup cooked quinoa
- 1 tablespoon fresh berries
- 1 tablespoon chopped nuts (almonds or walnuts preferred)
1 teaspoon chia seeds
1 teaspoon honey (or sugar)-no sweetener

Instructions:
1. Combine cooked quinoa and Greek yogurt in a mixing basin.
2. Garnish with fresh berries, almonds, and chia seeds.
3. To add sweetness, drizzle with honey or a sugar-free sweetener.

4. Combine thoroughly and serve a filling and nutritious quinoa breakfast dish.

3. Fruit and Cottage Cheese Parfait:

Ingredients:
- 1/2 cup cottage cheese (low-fat)
- 1/4 cup fresh fruit (sliced strawberries, blueberries, or peaches, for example)
1 tbsp. chopped nuts or granola
1 teaspoon honey (or sugar)-no sweetener

Instructions:
1. Layer the cottage cheese, fresh fruit, and chopped nuts or granola in a glass or bowl.
2. Drizzle with honey or a sugar substitute.
3. Gently mix or serve as a gorgeous layered parfait.

Remember to adapt ingredients and portion sizes based on your unique nutritional needs and blood sugar management goals. These breakfast alternatives have a balance of protein, healthy fats, and fiber-rich carbohydrates, which will help keep your blood sugar stable throughout the morning and provide you with sustained energy for the day ahead.

Experiment with various flavors, textures, and ingredients to find breakfast recipes that suit your taste buds and your lifestyle. You may start your day off well with a range of delicious and diabetic-friendly breakfast alternatives that will set the tone for a healthy and balanced meal plan.

Chapter 5

Lunch Recipes

Lunch is a great opportunity to fuel your body with the nutrition it needs to stay energized throughout the rest of the day. Diabetics benefit from lunch options that encourage blood sugar control, give satiety, and offer a variety of essential nutrients. In this section, we'll look at a variety of lunch options, including filling and delicious diabetic meals, nutritious and satisfying salad recipes, and hearty soups and stews for a satisfying midday meal.

1. Delicious and filling diabetic lunches:

a) Grilled chicken and vegetable skewers:
Ingredients:
- 4 ounces cubed skinless, boneless chicken breast - 1/4 cup diced bell peppers
- A single tablespoon of cherry tomatoes
- 1/4 cup chopped red onion

1 tablespoon olive oil - One tablespoon lemon juice
- 1 teaspoon dry herbs (thyme, rosemary) - Salt & pepper to taste

Instructions:
1. Turn up the heat on the grill or grill pan.
2. In a mixing bowl, stir the olive oil, lemon juice, dried herbs, salt, and pepper.
3. Skewer the red onion, cherry tomatoes, bell peppers, and cubes of chicken.
4. Brush the skewers with the marinade mixture.
5. Grill the skewers for 8 to 10 minutes, turning them over halfway through, or until the chicken is fully cooked and the vegetables are tender.
6. Include a salad or whole grain side dish with the grilled chicken and vegetable skewers.

b) Turkey lettuce wraps:
four large lettuce leaves, preferably romaine or iceberg; four ounces of lean ground turkey; and quarter cup of sliced bell peppers.
- 1/4 cup of cucumber slices - 2 tablespoons sliced red onion - 1 tablespoon tamari or

low-sodium soy sauce - 1 tablespoon rice vinegar - 1 tablespoon sesame oil
- Chopped nuts, sliced avocado, and a drizzle of hot sauce are available as garnishes.

1. In a nonstick skillet over medium heat, sauté the ground turkey until it is browned and well cooked.
2. Add the diced red onion, cucumber, and bell peppers; simmer for a few minutes, or until the vegetables are softened.
3. In a small bowl, combine the sesame oil, rice vinegar, and low-sodium soy sauce.
4. Evenly cover the turkey and vegetable combination in the skillet with the sauce.
5. Switch the heat off.
6. Place the lettuce leaves on a tray and top each with a layer of the turkey-vegetable mixture.
7. If desired, substitute additional toppings.
Serve these delectable turkey lettuce wraps by enclosing the filling with lettuce leaves.

2. Recipes for Healthy and Delicious Salads:

a) Salad with quinoa and grilled shrimp

Ingredients: 1 cup cooked quinoa, 2 cups mixed greens, and 4 ounces of deveined and peeled grilled shrimp.

- 1/4 cup cherry tomatoes, halved

- 1/4 cup diced cucumber

- 2 tablespoons of feta cheese that has been crushed;

Extra-virgin olive oil, 1 tablespoon

- Use salt and pepper to season as desired.

Instructions:

1. In a sizable mixing bowl, combine the cooked quinoa, mixed greens, cherry tomatoes, and diced cucumbers.

2. Add the feta cheese and grilled shrimp.

3. In a different small bowl, combine the lemon juice, olive oil, salt, and pepper.

4. Pour the dressing over the salad and toss to combine.

5. Offer the quinoa salad and grilled shrimp as a healthy and protein-rich lunch option.

b) Chicken Caesar Salad Ingredients:

- Sliced, grilled 4 ounces of chicken breast
- 2 cups chopped romaine lettuce
- 1/4 cup grated Parmesan cheese - 1/4 cup whole wheat croutons
- 2 tablespoons Caesar dressing (make your own or look for a brand with less sugar).
- Freshly ground black pepper, to taste

Instructions:

1. In a sizable mixing bowl, combine the chopped romaine lettuce, the grilled chicken slices, the grated Parmesan cheese, and the whole wheat croutons.

2. Dress the salad with the Caesar dressing by drizzling it over it and tossing to combine.

3. Taste-test and add freshly ground black pepper.

4. Indulge in a delicious and substantial Chicken Caesar Salad that is suitable for those with diabetes.

3. Hearty Soups & Stews for Lunch:

a) Soup with lentils and vegetables

Ingredients:
Olive oil, 1 tbsp 1 chopped tiny onion 2 minced garlic cloves 1 sliced carrot
- 1 celery stalk, chopped
- A cup of dried, rinsed lentils
- 4 cups low-sodium vegetable broth - 1 teaspoon of rosemary or thyme-flavored dry herbs
- Add salt and pepper to taste - Optionally garnish with fresh parsley

1. In a large pot, heat the olive oil to medium.
2. Add the celery, carrot, onion, and garlic. The vegetables should be softened in the sauté.
3. In a mixing dish, combine the lentils, vegetable broth, dried herbs, salt, and pepper.
4. After bringing the mixture to a boil, turn the heat down to low and simmer the lentils for 20 to 25 minutes, or until they are tender.
5. Check the seasoning and tweak it as necessary.
6. Pour the lentil and vegetable soup into bowls and, if desired, top with fresh parsley.

7. This hearty and nourishing soup is perfect for a satisfying and cozy meal.

b) Beef and vegetable stew:
Ingredients:
4 ounces of cubed lean beef, 1 tablespoon of olive oil, and 1 finely chopped tiny onion
- 2 minced cloves of garlic
- 1 sliced carrot - 1 celery stalk chopped
- 1 cup chopped fresh or canned tomatoes - 1 teaspoon dried thyme or rosemary - 2 cups low-sodium beef broth - Salt and pepper to taste
- Fresh parsley, chopped (optional) -

Instructions:
1. Heat the olive oil in a big saucepan or Dutch oven over medium heat.
2. Add the celery, carrot, onion, and garlic. The vegetables should be softened in the sauté.
3. In the skillet, brown the beef cubes on all sides.
4. Include the beef broth, diced tomatoes, dried herbs, and salt and pepper to taste.

5. Bring the mixture to a boil, then lower the heat and simmer the stew for one to one and a half hours, or until the meat is tender.
6. After tasting, adjust the seasoning to your liking.
7. If you'd like, garnish the meat and vegetable stew with finely chopped fresh parsley.
8. Use this hearty stew as a cozy lunchtime option.

Your midday meals will be intriguing and satisfying because of the range of flavors and textures in these lunch ideas. These recipes are made to offer balanced nutrition while maintaining your blood sugar levels, whether you prefer a filling and delectable diabetic lunch like grilled chicken and vegetable skewers or turkey lettuce wraps, a hearty soup or stew like vegetable and lentil soup or beef and vegetable stew, or any combination of the three.

The grilled shrimp and quinoa salad combines the protein-rich shrimp with the dietary fiber-rich quinoa and a variety of fresh veggies.

The light and tangy dressing gives this cool salad a taste boost. This traditional favorite is made up of creamy Caesar dressing, tender grilled chicken, crisp romaine lettuce, grated Parmesan cheese, and whole wheat croutons. You won't go to bed feeling hungry after this satisfying and well-rounded dinner.

Vegetable and lentil soup is a nutritious soup or stew option that is rich in fiber, vitamins, and minerals. Vegetables, lentils, and flavorful herbs come together to create a satisfying soup that is pleasant and filling. The beef and vegetable stew is a hearty and comfortable alternative if you prefer something more meaty. A hearty and flavorful stew that warms the body and the soul is made with tender meat, a variety of veggies, and aromatic spices.

These tasty and substantial lunch options are suitable for those with diabetes. By including a variety of products, flavors, and textures into your lunchtime routine, you may enjoy a balanced and healthful meal that promotes your overall health and diabetes management. Try out these recipes, make them your own by changing or adding ingredients to suit your preferences, and you'll soon discover new favorites you'll want to eat for years to come. Remember that making smart food decisions is the first step in leading a healthy lifestyle, and these recipes are meant to make that journey delicious and enjoyable.

Chapter 6

Dinner Recipes

As the day draws to a close, it's time to refuel your body with a hearty dinner that supports your diabetes diet while also satisfying your taste buds. We'll look at a variety of delectable and healthy dinner recipes in this section. Your evening meals will be excellent and suitable for diabetics thanks to these recipes, which include nourishing diabetic dinners, useful one-pot dishes, and vegetarian and vegan options.

1. Filling and flavorful diabetic dinners:

a) Baked salmon with lemon and herbs, using 1 tablespoon fresh lemon juice Salmon filet, 4 ounces, with 1 teaspoon olive oil, 1 teaspoon dry herbs (such as dill, thyme, or parsley), and optional lemon slices for garnish.

Turn the oven's temperature up to 400 degrees Fahrenheit (200 degrees Celsius).

2. Arrange the salmon filet on a baking sheet that has been lined with parchment paper.

3. Add some fresh lemon juice and olive oil to the fish.

4. Sprinkle the fish with the salt, pepper, and dry herbs evenly.

5. Bake the salmon for 12 to 15 minutes, or until it is well cooked and flakes easily.

6. Add lemon slices as a garnish, if preferred.

Serve the baked lemon herb salmon with steamed veggies or a mixed green salad for a balanced and flavorful supper.

b) A stir-fry dish with grilled chicken and vegetables

- 4 ounces sliced boneless, skinless chicken breast - 1 tablespoon low sodium soy sauce or tamari - 1 teaspoon sesame oil - 1 tablespoon rice vinegar

- 1 minced clove of garlic

- 1/2 teaspoon finely chopped fresh ginger

- 1 cup of a variety of veggies, such as bell peppers, broccoli, carrots, and snap peas.
1/9 cup olive oil
Add salt and pepper to taste. Garnishes are optional. sesame seeds or thinly chopped green onions

1. To make the marinade, combine in a small bowl the low-sodium soy sauce, rice vinegar, sesame oil, minced garlic, and grated ginger.
2. In a shallow dish, cover the cut chicken breast with the marinade. Give it a minimum of 15 minutes to marinate.
3. Heat the olive oil in a nonstick skillet or wok over medium-high heat.
4. Continue cooking until the marinated chicken is well cooked and browned.
5. Take the chicken out of the pan and set it on a platter.
6. In the same skillet, stir-fry the mixed vegetables until they are crisp and tender.
7. Combine everything in the skillet together with the cooked chicken.
8. Add salt and pepper as desired.

9. Serve the grilled chicken and vegetable stir-fry on its own or over a bed of cauliflower rice for a satisfying and delicious diabetic dinner.

2. One-Pot Dinners for Speedy Weeknight Meals:

a) Turkey and vegetable quinoa skillet:
Ingredients:
- 4 ounces of lean ground turkey - 1 tablespoon of olive oil - 1 minced garlic clove
- 1/2 cup chopped bell peppers
- 1/2 cup sliced zucchini - 1/2 cup tomatoes, diced
- 1 teaspoon dried herbs (like oregano or Italian seasoning) 1/2 cup cooked quinoa, to taste-seasoned with salt and pepper. - Optional garnishes include chopped fresh herbs or grated Parmesan cheese.

1. Heat the olive oil in a big pan over medium heat.

2. Continue cooking until the ground turkey is well-browned and cooked.

3. Take the turkey out of the pan and set it on a plate.

4. Include the minced garlic and onion in the same skillet. The onion should be cooked until translucent.

5. Add the diced tomatoes, zucchini, and bell peppers. Cooking vegetables until they are soft is recommended.

6. Combine the cooked quinoa with the cooked turkey in the skillet.

7. Taste-testing salt, pepper, and dried herbs.

8. To allow the flavors to meld, cook for a few more minutes.

9. If wanted, add grated Parmesan cheese and chopped fresh herbs to the turkey and vegetable quinoa dish as a garnish.

10. This one-pot meal is not only easy to make but also has a balanced amount of healthful grains, vegetables, and protein.

b) Shrimp and vegetable pasta: Ingredients:

- 1 tablespoon of extra virgin olive oil - 1 minced garlic clove - 4 ounces of whole wheat pasta - 4 ounces of peeled and deveined shrimp
- 1/2 cup chopped bell peppers
2 tablespoons of tomato sauce, 1/2 cup of halved cherry tomatoes, and 1/2 cup of sliced zucchini
- 1 tsp dry herbs, such as basil or oregano - Salt and pepper to taste - If preferred, garnish with finely chopped fresh basil or parsley

1. Prepare the whole-wheat pasta as directed on the package until it is al dente. Drain, then put aside.
2. Heat the olive oil in a big pan over medium heat.
3. Cook the minced garlic until it becomes fragrant.
4. In the skillet, sauté the shrimp until they are fully cooked and pink.
5. Take out and set aside the shrimp from the pan.
6. Add the zucchini slices, half of the cherry tomatoes, and diced bell peppers to the same

skillet. The vegetables should be softened in the sauté.

7. Combine the cooked shrimp in the skillet with the tomato sauce.

Add salt, pepper, and dried herbs as desired for seasoning.

9. Add the cooked pasta and combine the ingredients, coating the pasta with the sauce.

10. To allow the flavors to meld, cook for a few more minutes.

11. Fresh basil or parsley can be used as a garnish, if desired.

12. Serve the shrimp and vegetable spaghetti as a tasty, quick, and filling one-pot supper.

Dinner Options for Vegetarians and Vegans:

a) Curry with beans and vegetables:
Ingredients:
1 tablespoon coconut oil 1 small onion, diced 2 garlic cloves, minced

1 teaspoon curry spice - 1 tablespoon sliced fresh ginger - 1/2 teaspoon cumin powder - 1/2 teaspoon coriander powder

- Half a teaspoon turmeric - 1 cup chopped tomatoes

1 cup veggie broth 1 cup cooked lentils 1 cup mixed veggies (cauliflower, carrots, peas) - Season with salt and pepper to taste - Garnish with fresh cilantro (optional)

1. Preheat the coconut oil in a big skillet over medium heat.
2. Combine the chopped onion, minced garlic, and grated ginger in a mixing bowl. The onion should be clear after sautéing.
3. To the pan, add the curry powder, ground cumin, ground coriander, and turmeric. Stir the spices into the onion mixture thoroughly.
4. To the skillet, add the diced tomatoes and veggie broth. To mix, stir everything together.
5. Add the cooked lentils and mixed veggies and stir well.
6. Salt and pepper should be used to taste.

7. Lower the heat to a low setting and boil the curry for 15 to 20 minutes, or until the vegetables are tender and the flavors have melded.

8. Taste and fix the seasoning as needed.
9. Garnish the lentil and vegetable curry with fresh cilantro, if desired.
10. This vegan and vegetarian-friendly dinner choice has protein, fiber, and a variety of aromatic spices for a filling and delicious meal.

b) Stuffed Bell Peppers:
1 cup cooked quinoa - 1 cup cooked black beans - 1/2 cup diced tomatoes - 1/4 cup diced onion - 1/4 cup diced zucchini - 1/4 cup diced mushrooms
- 1/4 cup fresh or frozen corn kernels - 1/2 teaspoon cumin powder - 1/2 teaspoon pepper powder
- Season with salt and pepper to taste - Top with shredded vegan cheese or chopped fresh cilantro if desired

Instructions:

1. Set the oven's temperature to 375 degrees F (190 degrees C).

2. Combine the cooked quinoa, black beans, chopped tomatoes, onion, zucchini, mushrooms, and corn seeds in a mixing dish.

3. Stir in the ground cumin, chili powder, salt, and pepper. To mix, combine everything thoroughly.

4. Fill each bell pepper half halfway with the rice and veggie mixture, gently pressing it down.

5. Arrange the stuffed bell peppers on a parchment-lined baking pan.

6. Bake for 25-30 minutes, or until the bell peppers are soft and the edges are slightly browned.

7. Take the dish out of the oven and let it cool for a while.

8. If desired, garnish the stuffed bell peppers with shredded vegan cheese or chopped fresh cilantro.

9. These bright and fragrant stuffed bell peppers provide a delicious vegetarian or vegan supper option that is both nutritional and filling.

You have a wide range of choices with these supper preparations. Whether you prefer flavorful and wholesome diabetic dinners like baked lemon herb salmon or grilled chicken and vegetable stir-fry, easy one-pot meals like turkey and vegetable quinoa skillet or shrimp and vegetable pasta, or vegetarian and vegan-friendly options like lentil and vegetable curry or stuffed bell peppers, these recipes will satisfy your dietary needs while tantalizing your taste buds. Enjoy a tasty and diabetes-friendly dinner that nourishes your body and promotes general wellness.

Chapter 7

Appetizers and Snacks

It's essential to keep a variety of smart and diabetic-friendly snack and appetizer dishes on hand for when hunger strikes in between meals or you're hosting a party and want to serve some delicious appetizers. This section will look at a variety of meals that are both healthy and scrumptious, offering you satisfying choices to sate your cravings while maintaining a steady blood sugar level.

1. Diabetes Smart Snacking

a) Greek yogurt parfait
Ingredients:
- 1/2 cup Greek yogurt without added sugar
- One-fourth cup of mixed berries, such as blueberries, strawberries, and raspberries.
- One tablespoon of chopped nuts, either walnuts or almonds.

- Optional honey drizzle of 1 teaspoon - Optional cinnamon dusting

Instructions:
1. In a small bowl or glass, arrange the Greek yogurt, mixed berries, and chopped nuts.
2. To add a touch of sweetness, drizzle with honey, if desired.
3. Add cinnamon, if preferred, to enhance flavor.
4. Offer this nutrient-dense parfait, which is both hydrating and high in protein, as a full snack.

b) Veggie sticks covered with hummus:
- A variety of vegetable sticks (cucumber slices, carrot sticks, celery sticks, or bell pepper strips).
- 1/4 cup hummus, either handmade or bought

1. After washing the vegetables, slice or cut them into sticks.
2. Position the vegetable sticks on a dish for presentation.
3. Put hummus on the side to serve as a dip.
4. The combination of crunchy vegetables and creamy hummus makes this snack a delightful

and diabetic-friendly alternative. It is also full in fiber, vitamins, and minerals.

2. Tasty and Nutritious Diabetic-Friendly Snacks:

a) Baked zucchini fries
Ingredients: 1 medium zucchini cut into fries-like sticks; 1 tablespoon whole wheat breadcrumbs.
1/2 teaspoon dried herbs (oregano, basil) and two tablespoons of grated Parmesan cheese
- Toss in some olive oil and season as needed with salt and pepper.

Instructions:
Start by setting the oven's temperature to 425 degrees Fahrenheit (220 degrees Celsius).
2. In a mixing bowl, combine the whole wheat breadcrumbs, Parmesan cheese, dry herbs, salt, and pepper.
3. Lightly coat each zucchini stick with the breadcrumb mixture by dipping it into it.

4. Arrange the coated zucchini sticks on a baking sheet covered with parchment paper.
5. Lightly mist a can of olive oil spray onto the zucchini sticks.
6. Bake the zucchini fries in the oven for 15 to 20 minutes, or until crisp and golden.
7. Take the dish out of the oven and let it rest before serving.
8. Baked zucchini fries are a delicious, guilt-free alternative to normal french fries.

b) large button mushrooms with the stems removed.

1 cup chopped fresh spinach. 1/4 cup crumbled feta cheese. 1 minced garlic clove. 1 teaspoon olive oil. Use salt and pepper to your personal preference.

Instructions:
1. Set the oven's temperature to 375 degrees F (190 degrees C).
2. In a skillet over medium heat, warm the olive oil.

3. Cook the minced garlic until it becomes fragrant.

4. Include the spinach in the skillet and heat it through.

5. Take the pan from the heat and let it cool.

6. In a mixing dish, combine the cooked spinach, feta cheese, and salt and pepper.

7. Arrange the mushroom caps on a parchment-lined baking sheet.

8. Gently put the spinach-feta mixture into each mushroom cap with a spoon.

9. Bake for 15-20 minutes, or until the filling is fully cooked and the mushrooms are tender.

10. Take the dish out of the oven and let it cool for a while before serving.

11. A delicious and tasty appetizer that adds a healthy serving of greens to your snacking routine is stuffed mushrooms with spinach and feta.

3. Simple and speedy party appetizers

a) English cucumbers that have been chopped into rounds along with smoked salmon

- Smoked salmon, 4 ounces
- One teaspoon of cream cheese
- Fresh dill to garnish

On a serving platter, arrange the cucumber slices as desired and reserve.
2. Spread each slice of cucumber with a thin coating of cream cheese.
3. Top each slice of cucumber with a tiny piece of smoked salmon.
4. If preferred, garnish with fresh dill.
5. For parties or get-togethers, try these lovely cucumber nibbles with smoked salmon as an alternative to traditional appetizers.

b) Balsamic glaze is drizzled over cherry tomatoes, fresh mozzarella balls (bocconcini), and fresh basil leaves atop Caprese skewers.

Instructions:
1. Attach a cherry tomato, a chunk of fresh mozzarella, and a leaf of fresh basil to a skewer.
2. Continue by adding the remaining ingredients.
3. Place the caprese skewers in a serving dish.

4. Drizzle with balsamic glaze to increase flavor.
5. People love these caprese skewers because of the mouthwatering blend of flavors from the juicy tomatoes, creamy mozzarella, and fragrant basil.

With these snack and appetizer suggestions, you can choose from a wide range of sensible and delectable diabetic nutritional options. Whether you're looking for quick and simple snacks like Greek yogurt parfaits or veggie sticks with hummus, or you're planning a gathering and need savory appetizers like baked zucchini fries or spinach and feta stuffed mushrooms, these recipes are created to keep you satisfied and nourished while promoting your overall health and well-being. Graze on your treats!

Chapter 8

Dessert Recipes

Just because you're following a diabetic diet doesn't mean you have to give up delicious pleasures. In reality, there are lots of creative and delicious dessert options that you can eat while still controlling your blood sugar levels. This section will cover a variety of delectable dessert dishes that are suitable for diabetics. We'll also provide you with some practical baking advice and tricks.

1. Desserts suitable for diabetics:

a) Berry Chia Pudding recipe:
1 cup unsweetened almond milk (or any other non-dairy milk) and 2 teaspoons of chia seeds.
Unsweetened cocoa powder, 1 tablespoon
1 teaspoon of vanilla extract
- To taste, Stevia or your preferred sugar substitute - A variety of fresh berries (such as

strawberries, blueberries, or raspberries) for topping

Instructions:
1. In a mixing bowl, combine the almond milk, chia seeds, chocolate powder, vanilla extract, and sweetener.
2. Stir the mixture once more to remove any clumps after 5 to 10 minutes.
3. To allow the chia seeds to absorb the liquid and thicken the pudding, place the bowl in the refrigerator for at least two hours or overnight.
4. When it's time to serve, divide the chia pudding into serving glasses or bowls.
5. Add fresh berries as a garnish.
6. Use this creamy and nourishing berry chia pudding as a guilt-free treat to satiate your sweet tooth.

b) Apples with cinnamon baking:
Ingredients:
- 2 medium apples, such as Honeycrisp or Granny Smith

Unsalted butter, melted, 1 tablespoon 1 tablespoon of sugar substitute in granules
- 1/2 teaspoon ground cinnamon
- Chopped nuts and a dollop of unsweetened whipped cream are optional decorations.

1. Set the oven's temperature to 375 degrees F (190 degrees C).
2. Remove the apple cores and cut the apples in half horizontally.
3. In a small mixing bowl, combine the melted butter, sugar substitute, and ground cinnamon.
4. Arrange the apple halves on a baking sheet that has been lined with parchment paper.
5. Apply the melted butter mixture to the cut side of each apple half.
6. Bake the apples for 20 to 25 minutes, or until they are tender and just beginning to caramelize.
7. Take the baking sheet out and set it aside to cool somewhat.
8. If desired, cover the warm baked apples with unsweetened whipped cream, chopped nuts, or both.

9. These baked apples with cinnamon are a filling and diabetes-friendly dessert choice because to their delicious blend of toasted spices and natural sweetness.

2. Delicious desserts with a twist on health:

a) To make chocolate avocado flourless brownies, you'll need: two ripe avocados, peeled and pitted; half a cup of unsweetened cocoa powder.
- 1/2 cup granulated sugar replacement
- 2 eggs
- 1/4 teaspoon baking powder - 1 tablespoon almond flour - 1 teaspoon vanilla extract
- 1 dash of salt
- You can add chopped nuts or dark chocolate chips as decorations.

1. Set the oven's temperature to 350 fahrenheit (175 fahrenheit).
2. In a food processor, combine the avocados, chocolate powder, sugar substitute, eggs, and

vanilla extract. Blend the mixture until it's creamy and smooth.

3. Mix the almond flour, baking soda, and salt in a food processor. Once everything is well combined, pulse.

4. Spoon the batter into a parchment- or butter-lined baking pan.

5. Use a spatula to smooth the top and, if desired, garnish with chopped nuts or dark chocolate chips.

6. Bake the brownies for 20 to 25 minutes, or until the middle of a toothpick inserted into the center of the brownies comes out with a few moist crumbs.

7. Take out of the oven, let cool fully, then cut into squares.

8. These flourless chocolate avocado brownies are a delicious and healthier alternative to traditional brownies since the creamy avocado replaces the need for butter and almond flour is used in place of regular flour.

Greek yogurt parfait with berries:
Ingredients:

- 1 cup plain Greek yogurt
- 1 cup of mixed berries, including strawberries, blueberries, and raspberries.
two tablespoons of chopped nuts or granola -1 tablespoon of honey or sugar-optional sugar-free syrup
- Mint leaves, fresh, for garnish

Instructions:

1. In a glass or bowl, arrange Greek yogurt and mixed berries.
2. Sprinkle granola or chopped nuts on top to provide texture and crunch.
3. To add a hint of sweetness, sprinkle with honey or sugar-free syrup, if you'd like.
4. Garnish with fresh mint leaves to give color and freshness.
5. This light and protein-rich Greek yogurt berry parfait brings out the berries' inherent sweetness while providing a delectable and diabetes-friendly lunch.

3. Sugar-Free Baking Hints and Techniques:

a) Use natural sweeteners: To sweeten baked products without adding extra carbohydrates or increasing your blood sugar levels, use sugar alternatives such as stevia, erythritol, or monk fruit extract.

b) Experiment with alternative flours: Try substituting almond flour, coconut flour, or oat flour for refined wheat flour. These substitutes add a nice nuttiness, enhance fiber content, and have a less negative impact on blood sugar levels.

c) Incorporate fruits and vegetables: Use pureed fruits like applesauce or mashed bananas in your dishes as natural sweeteners and moisture enhancers. Grated zucchini or carrots can also provide moisture and nutrition to baked items.

d) Use spices to enhance flavors: Use spices such as cinnamon, nutmeg, vanilla essence, or almond extract to give depth and richness to your sugar-free treats.

e) Use portion control: Even sugar-free treats should be consumed in moderation. Maintaining regulated blood sugar levels and overall health requires paying attention to portion amounts.

You can indulge in tasty desserts without compromising your diabetes dietary objectives by exploring these dessert recipes and adopting sugar-free baking tips and tricks. From diabetic-friendly sweet snacks like berry chia pudding and baked apples with cinnamon to sumptuous sweets with healthy twists like flourless chocolate avocado brownies and Greek yogurt berry parfait, there are plenty of ways to satisfy your sweet taste while also supporting your health. Have fun creating and eating your guilt-free treats!

Chapter 9

Meal Plans and Sample Menus

Developing a well-rounded and balanced meal plan is critical to managing diabetes and living a healthy lifestyle. We will present you with a selection of meal plans and example menus made exclusively for diabetics in this section. These plans cater to various calorie levels, include seasonal and holiday variants, and offer tactics and advice for dining out while keeping to your dietary restrictions.

1. Weekly Meal Planning for Various Calorie Levels:

a) Meal Plan of 1,500 Calories:
- Breakfast: spinach and mushroom omelet with whole-grain toast - Snack: berries with Greek yogurt

- Grilled chicken salad with mixed greens, cherry tomatoes, cucumber, and balsamic vinaigrette for lunch
Carrot sticks with hummus for a snack - Baked salmon with quinoa and roasted asparagus for dinner - Sugar-free jello with whipped cream for dessert

b) Meal Plan of 1,800 Calories:
- Overnight oats with almond milk, chia seeds, and sliced almonds for breakfast
- Apple slices with peanut butter as a snack
- For lunch, make a turkey and avocado wrap with a whole-grain tortilla.
- Snack: Cream cheese-topped celery sticks
- Dinner: Stir-fried lean beef with broccoli, bell peppers, and brown rice
- For dessert, make a mixed berry smoothie with unsweetened almond milk.

c) Meal Plan of 2,200 Calories:
- Vegetable omelet with whole-grain bread and avocado for breakfast

- Snack: Greek yogurt with granola and mixed nuts
- Snack: hard-boiled eggs with slices of cucumber

Grilled chicken breast with sweet potato fries and steamed broccoli for dinner; dark chocolate-covered strawberries for dessert

2. Meal Plans for the Seasons and Holidays:

a) Summer Meal Plan: - Snack: Watermelon slices - Breakfast: Fresh fruit salad with Greek yogurt and a sprinkle of nuts
- Lunch: Skewers of grilled chicken or shrimp with grilled veggies
- Snack: Popsicles of frozen yogurt
- Grilled salmon with quinoa and grilled asparagus for dinner
- For dessert, grilled peaches with whipped cream.

b) Thanksgiving Menu:
- Breakfast: Pumpkin spice overnight oats - Snack: Cinnamon-spiced apple slices

- Roasted turkey breast with roasted Brussels sprouts and mashed cauliflower for lunch -
Roasted pumpkin seeds for snack
- Dinner: Herb-roasted chicken with almondine green beans and sweet potato casserole (using sugar alternatives)
- For dessert, make a sugar-free pumpkin pie with whipped cream.

3. Dining Strategies & Advice:

a) Plan ahead of time: Before you travel, look up the restaurant's menu online to locate diabetic-friendly selections. Rather of frying, choose for dishes that are grilled, baked, or steamed.

b) Choose lean proteins: Select lean cuts of meat such as grilled chicken, turkey, or fish. Dishes that are breaded or served with thick sauces should be avoided.

c) Watch portion sizes: To avoid overeating, order smaller quantities or share a meal with a dining companion. Request a takeout container and keep the leftovers for another meal.

d) Watch your carbohydrate intake: Avoid carbohydrate-rich foods like bread, pasta, and rice. Request substitutes such as more vegetables in place of starches.

e) Drink water or unsweetened beverages instead of sugary drinks: Instead of sugary drinks, drink water, unsweetened tea, or sparkling water with a touch of lemon or lime.

f) Don't forget about dessert: If you want to indulge in dessert, seek for low-sugar options or request fruit as a sweet finale to your dinner. You can also bring your own diabetic-friendly dessert to enjoy.

g) Communicate with your server: Inform your server of your dietary requirements and request any modifications or accommodations needed to accommodate your diabetes meal plan.

They might be able to give you more information or propose relevant options.

h) Avoid hidden sugars: Avoid sauces, dressings, and condiments that may contain hidden sugars. To enhance the flavor of your dish, request them on the side or use vinegar-based dressings, lemon juice, or herbs and spices.

i) Enjoy the dinner experience: Instead of focusing simply on the food, focus on the company and the enjoyment of the dining experience. To help control portion sizes and encourage better digestion, engage in conversation, taste the flavors, and eat slowly.

You may navigate restaurant menus with confidence, make informed choices that correspond with your diabetes meal plan, and yet enjoy the social part of dining out by following these dining out methods and ideas.

Remember that meal planning is a fluid process, and these sample meals are only a jumping-off point. Feel free to modify them according to your specific preferences, dietary limitations, and calorie requirements. Consult your healthcare physician or a qualified dietitian for individualized advice and to ensure that your meal plans are in line with your specific health objectives.

You may successfully navigate your diabetic diet while enjoying a range of delicious and healthy meals throughout the day and even on special occasions if you have these meal plans, sample menus, and dining out methods at your disposal. Good appetite!

Chapter 10

Managing Diabetes Through Lifestyle Choices:

Diabetes management entails more than just eating a healthy diet and taking medication. Lifestyle choices are important in managing your disease and promoting general well-being. In this section, we will look at major lifestyle aspects that can help you manage your diabetes, such as exercise and physical activity, stress management, and using diabetes information and support resources.

1. Diabetes Exercise and Physical Activity:

Regular physical activity and exercise are essential components of diabetes care. Physical activity improves insulin sensitivity, blood sugar control, weight management, the risk of cardiovascular problems, and overall health. Here are some key considerations:

a) Exercise Types: Include a mix of aerobic (brisk walking, cycling, swimming) and strength training (with weights or resistance bands) exercises in your regimen. Aim for at least 150 minutes a week of moderate-intensity aerobic activity, as well as strength training exercises twice a week.

b) Check with Your Healthcare Provider: Before beginning any fitness program, check with your healthcare provider to confirm it is safe and appropriate for your specific needs. Based on your health status and any current issues, they can provide specific advice and guidance.

c) Be Active Throughout the Day: Look for ways to be active throughout the day, such as taking short walks after meals, using the stairs instead of the elevator, or implementing stretching and movement breaks during inactive periods.

d) Regularly monitor your blood sugar levels before, during, and after exercise to ensure they stay within the desired range. Adjust your medication or food intake as needed to keep your blood sugar constant during physical activity.

e) Stay Hydrated: To avoid dehydration, drink lots of water before, during, and after exercise.

f) Maintain Consistency: Develop a regular exercise plan and strive for consistency. This will assist in developing a habit of physical activity and improving long-term diabetes management.

2. Diabetes and Stress Management:

Stress can have a substantial impact on blood sugar levels and diabetes management in general. Learning how to successfully manage stress is critical for sustaining good health. Consider the following approaches:

a) Recognize Stress Triggers: Recognize situations, events, or conditions in your life that cause stress. This insight can assist you in developing solutions to cope with such challenges.

b) Use Stress-Reduction Techniques: Deep breathing techniques, meditation, yoga, or mindfulness are all stress-relieving hobbies. These practices can aid in the relaxation of your mind and body, the reduction of stress hormones, and the promotion of emotional well-being.

c) Participate in Hobbies and Relaxation Activities: Make time for activities you enjoy and find calming, such as reading, listening to music, spending time in nature, or pursuing creative hobbies. These activities can be useful stress relievers.

d) Make Self-Care a Priority: Take care of your physical, mental, and emotional well-being. Make sure you're getting enough sleep, eating a healthy diet, and doing things that make you happy and relax.

e) Seek Help: Reach out to friends, family, or support groups to share your diabetes-related experiences, concerns, and feelings. Connecting with individuals who understand your situation can provide important support and encouragement.

f) Seek expert Help: If you find it difficult to handle stress on your own, consider obtaining help from a mental health expert who can provide guidance and stress management techniques.

3. Resources for Diabetes Education and Support:

Diabetes education and support are critical components of diabetes treatment success. Using educational resources and seeking help can help you make educated decisions, build self-management skills, and connect with a community of people going through similar experiences. Consider the following resources:

a) Enroll in diabetes education programs offered by healthcare facilities, community centers, or diabetic groups: These programs offer useful information on diabetes care, lifestyle changes, medication, and monitoring strategies. They may also provide diabetes instructors with lectures, workshops, or one-on-one consultations.

b) Support Groups: Join local or online support groups for people with diabetes. These communities provide a supportive environment in which you may share your experiences, trade tips and information, and receive encouragement from others who are going through similar difficulties. Connecting with individuals who understand your situation can provide emotional support as well as helpful insights.

c) Online Resources: Look into reliable diabetes education and support websites, blogs, and forums. These online resources frequently include a plethora of information, articles, meal plans, recipes, and lifestyle suggestions to help you manage your diabetes. However, make sure to use credible and evidence-based sources.

d) Diabetes applications: Use diabetes management applications to check blood sugar levels, medications, meals, and physical exercise. Some apps also include instructional information, reminders, and goal-setting capabilities to help you manage your diabetes.

e) Work closely with your healthcare team, which includes your doctor, diabetes educator, nutritionist, and pharmacist. They can provide you personalized advice, answer your questions, and keep track of your progress. Diabetes control requires regular check-ups and meetings with your healthcare team.

f) Diabetes Education Materials: Read diabetes-related books, periodicals, or newsletters. These materials can provide useful information about various elements of diabetes, such as nutrition, exercise, medication, and lifestyle changes.

Keep in mind that diabetes management is a continual process, and your requirements may change over time. Continue to be proactive in your search for information, support, and resources that correspond with your goals and interests. Adopting a comprehensive approach to diabetes treatment that includes physical activity, stress management, and access to educational resources will enable you to live a meaningful and balanced life while effectively controlling your diabetes.

Conclusion and Final Thoughts

Congratulations on finishing the pages of "Sugar-Free Success." Throughout this book, we've looked at several areas of diabetes management, such as a diabetic-friendly diet, lifestyle choices, and practical advice. Let us summarize some major aspects and offer encouragement and motivation for your ongoing journey as we complete this book.

1. Diabetes Understanding: We began by delving into the types, causes, and symptoms of diabetes, arming you with knowledge about this ailment. Understanding diabetes is the first step toward regaining control of your health and making sound decisions.

2. diabetes-Friendly Diet: We addressed key tools and ingredients for diabetes cooking, outfitted your kitchen with appropriate equipment, and highlighted the must-have diabetic pantry products. By stocking your kitchen with the necessary tools and supplies, you will be well-equipped to produce delicious and nutritious meals that will benefit your health.

3. Basics of Diabetic Meal Planning: We covered the fundamentals of diabetic meal planning, such as portion control and carbohydrate counting, and stressed the significance of constructing a balanced plate. These tactics help you maintain stable blood sugar levels by ensuring that your meals are well-balanced and satisfying.

4. Breakfast, Lunch, Dinner, Snack, and Dessert Recipes: For each mealtime, we supplied a variety of recipes, including invigorating breakfast options, nourishing lunches, delectable dinners, smart snacking ideas, and diabetic-friendly sweets. While keeping your diabetes control goals in mind, these meals provide diversity, flavor, and nutrition.

5. Meal Plans and Sample Menus: We included weekly meal plans for various calorie levels, seasonal and holiday meal plans, and eating out tactics. These materials provide structure and inspiration, making it easier and more flexible to prepare your meals.

6. Diabetes Management Through Lifestyle Choices: We discussed the significance of exercise and physical activity, stress management, and the use of diabetes education and support resources. You can improve your overall well-being and effectively manage your diabetes by implementing these lifestyle changes into your everyday routine.

Finally, managing diabetes is a lifelong endeavor that involves dedication, understanding, and self-care. Remember that everyone's journey is different, so it's critical to listen to your body, collaborate with your healthcare team, and make modifications based on your own needs.

I want to support and motivate you as you embark on this path. Living with diabetes might be difficult at times, but remember that you are not alone. Seek help from loved ones, medical professionals, and diabetes groups. Share your stories, ask questions, and seek advice and encouragement from others.

As you adjust to your new lifestyle, be patient and nice to yourself. Diabetes management is an ongoing learning process, with ups and downs along the way. Celebrate your victories, no matter how minor, and learn from your setbacks. Every day is a new chance to make better choices and take steps toward improved health.

Remember that you have the ability to manage your diabetes and live a lively, fulfilling life. You are well-equipped to manage your diabetic path with confidence if you use the knowledge, techniques, and recipes presented in this book, as well as the support of your healthcare team and loved ones.

Accept this new chapter with hope and determination. Maintain your commitment to your health by making educated decisions and prioritizing self-care. You are empowering yourself to live a vibrant life and thrive despite the challenges of diabetes by doing so.

I wish you success, good health, and a tasty voyage ahead!

9 798395 164575